Yoga & Progressive Relaxation Response

Before Transcendence - Savasana & Beyond

By Vie Binga & Tim Ganley

Dedication

To all those out there who need Savasana the most....

- Vie &

Tim

Acknowledgments

We would like to thank all of our Teachers, through the years, official and unofficial, who showed us the way to a deeper understanding.

This work would have never happened without, in particular, the direct teachings of Prof. R.H. Singh and Vasant Lad, and the influence of Steven Kotler, David Asprey and Dr. Herbert Benson.

- Vie & Ti

Preface

The little classroom clock sitting on the bookshelf shows 6:47 p.m. on a Monday evening. The 55-min class started at 6:00 p.m. sharp, as always.

"And now please, lie on your back for the best part of your practice, where you get to absorb all the amazing benefits."

The above phrase, has through the years, almost always been our Clients' and Students' most favorite part. It marks the beginning of savasana, or corpse pose. Now you are thinking one of two things: "well of course, this is their favorite part, they do not have to do anything, they are just lying there." Yes, you are correct in your observation. If on the other hand you are a strong type a personality, you are telling yourself: "what a waste that part is, I would never stay in the room, let alone pay some one to have me lying on the floor doing nothing for minutes at a time. Yes, you are also correct in your observation, notice the "almost always" terminology in the beginning of this paragraph.

Both of the above remarks demonstrate that savasana is one of these very misunderstood and at the same time underestimated poses of a yoga practice. This is the reason we decided to dedicate a whole eBook to it. We had initially wanted to name it "In Defense Of Savasana". But after talking with several people, and conducting a reader poll between 2 main possible titles, we decided to go with the general consensus instead.

We believe that savasana is a lot more than a pose; savasana is an integral part of a yoga class. In fact, if performed properly, savasana should be part of any physical exercise session.

This eBook explores all the forgotten why's and how's of the infamous corpse pose. No prior knowledge or experience is required or assumed.

After reading this book, we guarantee that you will have all the tools you need to guide yourself and/or your class through the most effective and efficient savasana part heavenly possible.

We always love to hear back from our readers on what the book's biggest influence on them was. Let us know yours!

Thank you for reading!

- Vie & Tim, January, 2016

Introduction

How You Can Receive Everything By Doing Nothing

Have you ever wondered what the difference between action and doing is?

A quick dictionary search shows results such as:

"Doing is the activities in which a particular person engages."

"Action is the fact or process of doing something, typically to achieve an aim."

"As nouns the difference between action and doing is that action is something done so as to accomplish a purpose while doing is a deed or action, especially when somebody is held responsible for it."

The common denominator to all of the above is that action is purpose driven, where doing is activity based.

In today's world, we are conditioned to think, even believe, that doing is the only way to move forward, achieve something greater than we already have, become something greater than we already are. We tend to be activity driven and confuse doing with action. We have even been infected by the epidemic of multitasking.

Modern neuroscience and neuropsychology research shows not only that multitasking is actually harming our brain and our performance but in reality, non-doing is a lot of times the most effective and efficient form of action.

Action does not take place unless we have created space for it, whether that be physical, mental or emotional. The only way to create space is by stopping. Stopping whatever it is that we are consumed in doing.

How many times have you found your keys or something else you misplaced, after you stopped looking for it?

How many times have you remembered the name of a song, or a place after you stopped trying to recall it?

How many times have you had an inspiring idea after "wasting time" during a small talk with a friend?

We are by no means advocating "laziness". What we are saying, is that our bodies, our emotions and our minds, just like everything else in life, need a break, in order to repair themselves from the daily, constant wear and tear. When that break is given to them purposefully, with the right intention and at the right time and place, wonders can happen.

Below is an excerpt from an interview with Josh Davis, Ph.D. Director of Research and Lead Professor for the NeuroLeadership Institute on mind-wandering and what it can do for our mental productivity.

"Let your mind wander for a few minutes and then come back to it. That's something that often is a little counterintuitive for people but it's something that probably everyone will have done at some point in their life and can recognize.... That has psychological benefits that are very hard to get otherwise. Some of the things that happen when our minds wander is that we integrate certain neural networks that are involved in what we call executive functions or which have to do with things like staying focused on a goal and holding ideas in mind... Another thing mind-wandering does it helps with creative incubation so that's when you've been working on a challenge. Creative it can be, design type of creative but can also be creative in many ways. Maybe you're trying to figure out what's the right theme to put on a certain project. Anything that's really complex is going to have some creative element. You've been working on a creative challenge if you then mind-wander and come back to it. You're more likely to come up with creative solutions and the solutions you come up with are going to be rated as more creative than if you hadn't, than if you had just spent that same amount of time working on it."

The same principles of non-action apply to the physical and emotional level as the following excerpt from Dr. Herbert Benson's work states.

"Stress does not cause pain, but it can exacerbate it and make it worse. Much of chronic pain is 'remembered' pain. It's the constant firing of brain cells leading to a memory of pain that lasts, even though the bodily symptoms causing the pain are no longer there. The pain is residing because of the neurological connections in the brain itself."

We are not asking you to take our word for it. What we ask is that you take action and find out for yourselves.

How To Use This Book

This book is intentionally written in such a way that it can be read cover to cover, and readily implemented. If you are reading it as a practitioner, all you need is your mat. If you are reading it as a Teacher, all you need is at least one Student.

We are starting by lying down our definition of the savasana process so we are all on the same wavelength. We then proceed through every step of the way, narrating the class as if you were present. We give warning of some common pitfalls and we reinforce good habits.

In the FAQ section we take the time to address the most common questions we have gotten through the years.

"If you are anxious, you can't learn. It's like dropping seeds on concrete. With a quiet mind, people take things in." -*Dr. Herbert Benson*

Are you ready?

What Is Savasana?

Savasana is the Sanskrit word for the Corpse posture. Lie on your back, with the legs extended, feet apart, arms a few inches away from the rest of the body, palms facing up or down.

Savasana is some times also spelled Shavasana. For the sake of simplicity, in this book, we are going to be using the term savasana. If you are interested in the Sanskrit language and in all the transliteration details, you can start by referring to the suggested Wikipedia link in the Bibliography section or look up the work of one of my teachers, Nicolai Bachman, also referenced in the Bibliography section.

According to Prof. R. H. Singh, the Corpse Pose is the most popular among the relaxation postures. It is not a meditation posture, however. Meditation and relaxation are closely interrelated processes. The aim of the Corpse Pose is muscular and mental relaxation, not sleep or meditation. Sitting postures are the ones conducive to meditation, not lying down.

According to David Coulter, relaxation in yoga, means lying down in savasana and relaxing from head to toe. Meditation is a stage beyond. Relaxation releases deep tensions and meditation pulls the mind inward and introduces it to higher states. Meditation cannot begin without a relaxed body, mind and emotional state.

The fact that savasana is a relaxation pose does not imply that it is easy. Old injuries and hidden tension can make this posture increasingly irritating. Have you ever wondered why most people like to sleep curled up on their sides? Has your mind ever been able to wander while your lower back is "killing" you?

Having taught Yoga and several other forms of Fitness for decades, we learned that savasana is better implemented as a process instead of as a posture.

By preparing accordingly, yourself as a practitioner or your Students as a Teacher, it is guaranteed that the benefits will be multifold.

"Beware the barrenness of a busy life." - *Socrates*

When To Do Savasana?

We have found that the most practical way to incorporate savasana into a yoga session and / or any physical exercise session is at the very end. The main reasons are the following:

- ☐ The Students are more willing to "lie down" and quiet their bodies and minds after they feel that they indeed accomplished something.
- ☐ The Students are more likely to let their mind wander, hence relax, instead of worrying how well they are going to perform in class.
- ☐ It gives the Students' bodies, minds and emotions the chance to absorb all the neurophysiological benefits of the session that preceded.

We recommend that you adjust the flow of the class and physically and mentally prepare the Students with Breathing Exercises before savasana. You only need to take 2-5 minutes.

There are several different exercises that you can choose from. The most important one is Belly Breathing. The reason being, this is the technique you want them to focus on during the actual Final Relaxation part.

Belly Breathing

You can have them practice Belly Breathing while seated, either in easy sitting or rock pose (aka hero's pose.)

Recommended Verbiage

- Place your left hand on your belly and your right hand on your chest.

- ☐ Exhale through your nose; letting as much air out of your lungs as you can and notice how your belly goes in, in other words it shrinks like a balloon.

- ☐ Now inhale through your nose, allowing as much air into your lungs as you can and notice how your belly goes out, in other words, it expands like a balloon.

- ☐ Try to keep your chest from moving. The less your chest moves and the more your belly expands and shrinks (i.e. the more you engage the abdominal muscles), the fuller your breathing becomes.

After about 4 rounds, you are ready to prepare your room for savasana.

Tip #1

This is the type of breathing you want to be using for the most part during your day (excluding times of breathing exercises, strenuous activity, etc.)

Tip #2 - For Teachers

While your Students are practicing belly breathing, remind them that this is the type of breathing they want to be using for the most part during their day; If they have ever watched a baby breathe, this is how their belly moves.

Preparation For Savasana

Preparing The Room

One of the two most equally important parts during the final relaxation is that the Students feel safe and comfortable.

For them to feel safe, you need to make sure that the room is secure. Please, go through the following checklist and adjust accordingly for your location and circumstances.

- ☐ Lock the door, so you do not have people randomly walking in.

- ☐ Adjust the temperature and air flow so that it is comfortable for every one.

- ☐ Turn off the lights, or at least dim them enough.

- We choose not to play music in our classes but if you wish to, adjust the type and volume accordingly. If the outside noise is too disturbing, you may wish to consider some type of white noise for inside the room.

Please, keep in mind that when it comes to temperature, air flow, lighting and sound, you will never be able to fully please every one. The best course of action is:

- Become aware of all the classroom parameters.
- Decide on what needs to be adjusted for the benefit of your Students.
- Make a conscientious effort along those lines.
- If a Student is not happy with the circumstances, do not take it personal.

Preparing Yourself As A Teacher

In the previous section, we wrote, "one of the two most equally important parts during the final relaxation is that the Students feel safe and comfortable." You must be wondering what the other part is. The other part is You as the Teacher.

You must both *create* and *hold* the space for them to be able to relax. Believe it or not, we have found that *holding* the space is the hardest part for a Teacher.

What To Do

- [ ] After you have taken care of the room preparation, sit quietly in your easy sitting, at the front of the room facing your Students.
- [ ] Keep your spine erect and stay still as if you are getting ready for meditation.

- ☐ Focus at your belly breathing, keeping your eyes open.
- ☐ Keeping your eyes open allows you to notice any discomfort that your Students may be experiencing while lying down, such as back pain or hip pain. This will help improve your teaching methodologies.
- ☐ Resist the urge of drinking water, adjusting your clothes, fixing your hair, toweling off your hands or face, fidgeting, clearing your throat, responding to an itch, shuffling paper, etc.
- ☐ Stay seated and still, holding the sacred space for your Students relaxation response to occur.

Preparing The Students

This is the part where you invite the Students to, please, lie on their back for the best part of their practice, where they get to absorb all the amazing benefits.

Recommended Verbiage

- ☐ Please, lie on your back, feet towards me, for the best part of your practice, where you get to absorb all the amazing benefits.
- ☐
- ☐ Separate your legs to the width that makes your lower back happy.
- ☐ Bring your arms a few inches away from the rest of your body.
- ☐ Turn your palms to face the ground or the sky, whichever way feels best on your shoulders.
- ☐ Close your eyes.

Tip #1

Some yoga traditions consider it being disrespectful to the Teacher when the Students feet face him or her. Therefore, they recommend that during savasana the Students turn around so their head lies towards the Teacher. We believe every part of the body to be equally sacred, hence we do not recommend that you do or encourage that. However, it is something you may want to keep in mind if you visit certain yoga centers or ashrams in the future.

Tip #2

If it is uncomfortable for you to lie on your back as instructed, please modify accordingly. You can always bend your knees, bring your arms on your chest, roll up your towel and set it underneath your head, etc.

Tip #3 - For Teachers

As an instructor, please, do not force your Students into the "exact" Corpse Pose. Old injuries and hidden tension may make it counter productive or even injurious for them.

Tense& Release

The neurophysiology and scientific explanations are well beyond the scope of this eBook. However, we are going to highlight certain bullet items that you can use in your own research, should you wish to delve deeper into the subject of the Progressive Relaxation Response.

☐ Contraction and relaxation are the normal functions of skeletal muscles.

☐ The motor neurons are what makes our musculoskeletal system contract and relax.

☐ Everyone has a resting level of muscle tension. Some people have a great amount of tension at rest, others less. When people are under acute stress, their muscles tend to have higher levels of resting tension that can be painful and fatiguing.

☐ The relaxation response is defined as our ability to make our body release chemicals and brain signals which make our muscles and organs slow down, thereby increasing blood flow to the brain.

☐ The progressive relaxation response, through tense and release teaches us how to silence our motor neurons.

☐ After you tense and relax muscles, the tension level not only returns to the original level, but also will automatically drop below the original level, producing even greater relaxation to the muscles.

Tense & Release Verbiage

We recommend that you use the Abbreviated Version when you do not have enough time for the Full Version. It is best to use this short version than completely skip the Tense & Release. Having said that, you are of course more than welcome to use either technique any time you wish.

Abbreviated Version

- ☐ We are going to do 3 sets of total body Tense and Release.

- ☐ When I ask you to inhale you are going to take a breath in, lifting your whole body except the glutes an inch or so of the ground tensing as much as you can. You can even make fists and squeeze your whole face towards your nose.

- ☐ When I ask you to exhale, you are going to breath out releasing everything on the ground.

- ☐ Inhale and lift. Tense, tense, tense, make fists, face to the nose. (This is the 1st time.)
- ☐ Exhale, release.

- ☐ Inhale and lift. Squeeze, squeeze, squeeze. (This is the 2nd time.)
- ☐ Exhale, release.

- ☐ Last time. Lift; tense everything as much as you can. (This is the 3rd time.)
- ☐ And exhale, release.

The above verbiage takes about a minute or so, on average. You are now ready to move straight to the Relaxation Verbiage in the next section.

Full Version

We are going to do our individual Tense & Releases.

- ☐ When I name a muscle group your are going to take a breath in, raise it an inch or so off the ground, tense it as much as you can and on an exhale you are going to release it back to the ground.

- ☐ Right leg, an inch off the ground, tense, tense, tense.
- ☐ Exhale, release.

- ☐ Other leg, an inch off the ground, tense, tense, tense.
- ☐ Exhale, release.

- ☐ Right arm, raise it an inch off the ground, make a tight fist, tense, tense, tense, point all the fingers, spread the hand as much as you can.

☐ Exhale, release.

☐ Other arm, raise it an inch off the ground, make a tight fist, tense, tense, tense, point all the fingers, spread the hand as much as you can.

☐ Exhale, release.

☐ Inhale and lift your glutes an inch off the ground. Squeeze them as much as you can. Tense, tense, tense.

☐ Exhale, release.

☐ Inhale and make your belly as big as you can, like a balloon.

☐ Exhale, release.

☐ Inhale and keeping your head on the ground, get the chest and shoulders off the ground. Tense, tense, tense.

☐ Exhale, release.

- ☐ Inhale and squeeze your whole face towards the nose. Make the tightest face you can. Squeeze, squeeze, squeeze.
- ☐ Exhale, release.

- ☐ Inhale, open your eyes, stick your tongue out, look back, stretch your face as much as you can.
- ☐ Exhale, release.

The above verbiage takes about two minutes or so, on average. You are now ready to move straight to the Relaxation Verbiage in the next section.

Tip #1

It does not matter whether you start from the right leg or the left leg. It is a good practice to periodically switch and not only start on the same side all the time.

Tip #2 - For Teachers

It is really important that you raise and lower your voice accordingly, in order to emphasize the *tensing* part of the action and the *releasing* part of the action. This is also the reason that the tension promoting cues are repeated three times. It encourages the Students to fully implement both phases.

Final Relaxation

It is very important to guide yourself and / or your Students in a sequential, step by step manner through all the different body parts. Avoid jumping for example from the knees to the shoulders or vice versa.

Recommended Verbiage

- ☐ Relax your toes.
- ☐ Relax your feet.
- ☐ Relax your ankles.
- ☐ Relax your calves.

- ☐ All tension is going away from your knees.
- ☐ All tension is going away from your thighs.
- ☐ All tension is going away from your hips.

- ☐ Release all tension from your glutes.
- ☐ Release all tension from your back.

- ☐ Relax your fingers.

- ☐ Relax your hands.
- ☐ Relax your wrists.
- ☐ Relax your forearms.

- ☐ All tension is going away from your elbows.
- ☐ All tension is going away from your arms.

- ☐ Release all tension from your belly.
- ☐ Release all tension from your chest.
- ☐ Release all tension from your shoulders.
- ☐ Release all tension from your neck.

- ☐ Relax your jaw.
- ☐ Release your tongue from the roof of your mouth.
- ☐ Relax your forehead.

- ☐ Relax your face.
- ☐ Relax your body.

- ☐ You are completely relaxed.
- ☐ Your body is completely relaxed.

- ☐ You are completely relaxed. (You are repeating for the second time, not a typo. :-))
- ☐ Your body is completely relaxed.

- ☐ You are completely relaxed. (You are repeating for the third time, not a typo. :-))
- ☐ Your body is completely relaxed.

- ☐ For the next couple of minutes, bring your attention to the spot below your belly button and keeping your eyes closed and your focus there, just breathe.

The above verbiage takes about a minute and a half or so, on average.

Tip #1

The relaxation verbiage ends by guiding the practitioner to bring their attention "to the spot below the belly button". This area is also known as the second chakra, in the Yogic Tradition, or the hara area, in the Japanese Tradition. It is believed to be the container of our most vital and creative energy. Regardless of any esoteric meanings, by guiding the practitioner to bring their attention to that area, you are assisting them in grounding themselves, by focusing within their body, and away from their head.

Tip #2 - For Teachers

Keep your voice soft but not too soft. You still want to be firm, assertive and heard comfortably by every one in the room. There is nothing relaxing about some one having to struggle, trying to hear the Teacher.

Coming Out Of Savasana

It is very important that you bring yourself and/or your class out of savasana in a very gentle manner. We have seen Students literally rock up into the seated position right after savasana. This habit neurophysiologically undoes all the benefits gained during the session that preceded.

The most effective way to come out of savasana is to go back into our one and only life-long possession, our breath. In fact, Savasana, in the Yogic Tradition is described as symbolizing the process of rebirth.

Recommended Verbiage

☐   Feel your belly rise as you inhale and sink as you exhale.

- [ ] Feel your toes and your fingers, your ankles and your wrists. Make small movements.

- [ ] On an inhale, raise your arms up over your head, on the ground behind you and extend. Extend your left side, extend your right side, extend both sides making your spine as long as you can.

- [ ] On an exhale, hug your knees towards your chest, gently rocking from side to side massaging your lower back.

- [ ] Roll over to your right side, in your fetal position, take a moment there, and slowly, using both arms for support, push yourself up into the easy sitting.

- [ ] Thank you all so much for being here today. You have a wonderful rest of the day. Namaste!

For those of you teaching group classes where the mats may be closer than typical, here is an equally beneficial way to come out of savasana that keeps people within their mat at all times. So, no chance of any one's hands touching some one else's toes.

Recommended Verbiage

- ☐ Feel your belly rise as you inhale and sink as you exhale.

- ☐ Feel your toes and your fingers, your ankles and your wrists. Make small movements.

- ☐ On an inhale, hug your knees towards your chest, gently rocking from side to side massaging your lower back.

- ☐ On an exhale, roll over to your right side, in your fetal position, take a moment there, and slowly, using both arms for support, push yourself up into the easy sitting.

☐ When you are up into the easy sitting, on an inhale raise both arms over your head and on an exhale bring your left hand on the ground by your left hip leaning to the left so you are fully extending your right side.

☐ Inhale both arms up again and on an exhale, repeat on the opposite side.

☐ Now, inhale both arms up, interlace the fingers, turn the palms to face the sky and make your spine as tall as you can, keeping the shoulders down and away from the ears.

☐ On an exhale, bring the hands to the heart center, Thank you all so much for being here today. You have a wonderful rest of the day. Namaste!

Tip #1

It does not matter which side you turn to when going into your fetal position, it can be right or left. It is a good practice to periodically switch and not only use one side all the time.

Tip #2 - For Teachers

In order to keep your class uniform and hence comfortable, be specific as of to which side the Students should turn to, when guiding them to go into their fetal position. This way, they do not end up facing each other. So, it is not recommended to use cues such as "roll over into your favorite side."

Tip #3 - For Teachers

It is more important than you realize to be extremely punctual about ending your class on time (beginning as well.) Your Students have meetings to attend, children to pick up, errands to run, planes to catch, etc. They have planned their day expecting the class to end at a certain time. Taking the class past that time for a few extra minutes of savasana, will be not only counter productive, it could even be extremely stressful to them. It is your responsibility as a Teacher to respect your Students' time and energy.

Frequently Asked Questions

Q. I have heard some people say that you are not supposed to fall asleep during savasana. Is that true?

A. Savasana is not a meditative pose. Savasana is a relaxation pose that prepares you for meditation. Relaxation is when you allow your mind to "wander" in order for your nervous system to prepare for meditation. So, even though falling asleep is not recommended or even desired, it is not considered a "bad" thing. If it happens once in a while, it is ok, let it go. If it happens on a regular basis, we recommend that you start addressing diet and lifestyle that may be affecting your health.

Q. How long should savasana be? Some people say half hour, is that correct?

A. There are many anecdotal answers to this question. There is not enough scientific evidence to suggest one vs. the other. Some traditions say half hour, Prof. R.H. Singh suggests 20 minutes twice a day, Baron Baptiste teaches a 7-minute savasana. Dr. Herbert Benson suggests 10-20 minutes of progressive muscle relaxation response practice.

As explained in the beginning sections, the process of savasana that is described in this eBook is the most effective and efficient method of relaxation that can be implemented in any physical exercise session for personal use and for teaching group classes. It combines both the corpse pose (from the Yogic Tradition) and the progressive muscle relaxation response (from modern neurophysiological research.)

Q. Have you had students who just walked out of the room during savasana?

A. As a matter of fact, no. You as the Teacher need to take control of the class and set the parameters before hand. The process that we follow is that if a Student lets us know that they need to leave a few minutes early, we ask that they leave extremely quietly before the savasana session starts, during breath-work for example. We make sure that their departure takes place seamlessly by even unlocking the door for them and locking it again.

Q. In some classes, I have seen teachers read inspirational passages to students during savasana, placing essential oils on their forehead, stretching their necks and legs, in other words catering to them in some lovely ways. Why don't you mention that in this book?

A. Yes, yes, and yes, as in they are all wonderful techniques. However, their purpose is different from the purpose of our savasana process. Since this is a question that comes up a lot, actually it is 3 questions in 1; we will give you the quick version of why they are different than our savasana.

A1. Reading during savasana, such as in a guided meditation or visualization exercise, takes away from the mind-wandering and daydreaming aspects that we are targeting.

A2. Essential oils, such as in aromatherapy, may cause discomfort for Students sensitive or allergic to certain scents, which would be counter-productive to the relaxation process. Asking the class ahead of time for whoever does not wish to experience the essential oil, to raise their hand, is pointless. The smell spreads; the Students who do not like the smell simply won't come back.

A3. "Touching" Students in a class, is a very "touchy" subject, pun intended. Touching may bring up a whole lot of past psychological and emotional issues that the Student and the Teacher are not ready to address. Asking the class ahead of time for whoever does not wish to be touched, to raise their hand, does not guarantee that it will work. Students often are hesitant to speak up since they do not want to feel singled out, they simply won't come back.

Q. Do you have to practice the Corpse Pose at the end?

A. Absolutely not. According to certain Yogic Traditions, the Corpse Posture is even practiced in between other poses or even in the beginning. We have found that in today's context, it is more appealing to the Students, hence more practical, if it is performed at the end of the session.

Epilogue

"One of the symptoms of an approaching nervous breakdown is the belief that one's work is terribly important."

~Bertrand Russell (British philosopher, logician, mathematician, historian, writer, social critic and political activist)

The most common excuse we have heard from people of all disciplines is that they don't have time for relaxation. The moment you think that you don't have time for it, is the moment that you need it the most. This is the reason we designed savasana as an only 6-8 minute long process that combines all the physical, mental and emotional benefits of the Yogic Tradition and modern neurophysiological research. You will be extremely surprised at how much mental focus and physical energy you are going to have after a properly implemented savasana.

The only missing link between You and Your Renewed Self is You Taking Action.

About the Authors

Vie Binga is a lifestyle entrepreneur, outdoor adventurer and author. She loves to biohack blending science and nature, to enhance physical and mental performance, sharing her findings with others. She believes that high intention, sincere effort, and intelligent execution will always make an impact in people's lives and the world. When she is not teaching or writing, she can be found rock climbing, surfing, whitewater kayaking or scuba diving.

Tim Ganley is a lifestyle entrepreneur, outdoor adventurer and author. He loves experimenting with disciplines that lead to physical and mental strength and endurance. He believes that if people learn about the state of flow and practice building their life around it, the world will be much happier. When he is not teaching or designing new programs, he can be found white water kayaking, rock climbing, scuba diving, off road biking or surfing.

We would love to hear from you!

Training@asktimandvie.com

Instagram: @ask_tim_and_vie

Periscope: @ask_tim_and_vie

Twitter: @ask_tim_and_vie

Bibliography

1) <u>Anatomy of Hatha Yoga by H. David Coulter (2001)</u>

2) <u>Body-Mind-Spirit Integrative Medicine in Ayurveda Yoga & Nature Care by Prof. R. H. Singh (2009)</u>

3) <u>The Language of Yoga: Complete A to Y Guide to Asana Names, Sanskrit Terms, and Chants by Nicolai Bachman</u>

4) <u>The Rise Of Superman: Decoding the Science of Ultimate Human Performance by Steven Kotler</u>

5) <u>The Wellness Book: The Comprehensive Guide to Maintaining Health and Treating Stress-Related Illness, Herbert Benson, MD.</u>

6) https://www.bulletproofexec.com/josh-davis-chill-out-daydreamthe-multitasking-myth270/

7) https://www.psychologytoday.com/blog/the-neuroscience-mindfulness/201601/the-myth-multitasking

8) https://nccih.nih.gov/health/stress/relaxation.htm

9) https://en.m.wikipedia.org/wiki/Shavasana